The
CAVEMAN
CLEANSE

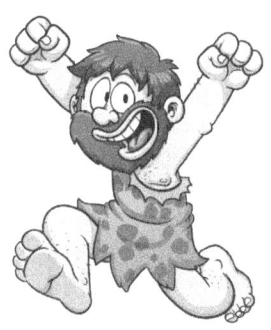

BY LEAH BELL

ISBN-13: 978-1522952664
ISBN-10: 1522952667

"Having clear skin gives you the confidence to be who you truly are. It's about being free in your own skin, not trapped in it." **—Leah Bell**

Table of Contents

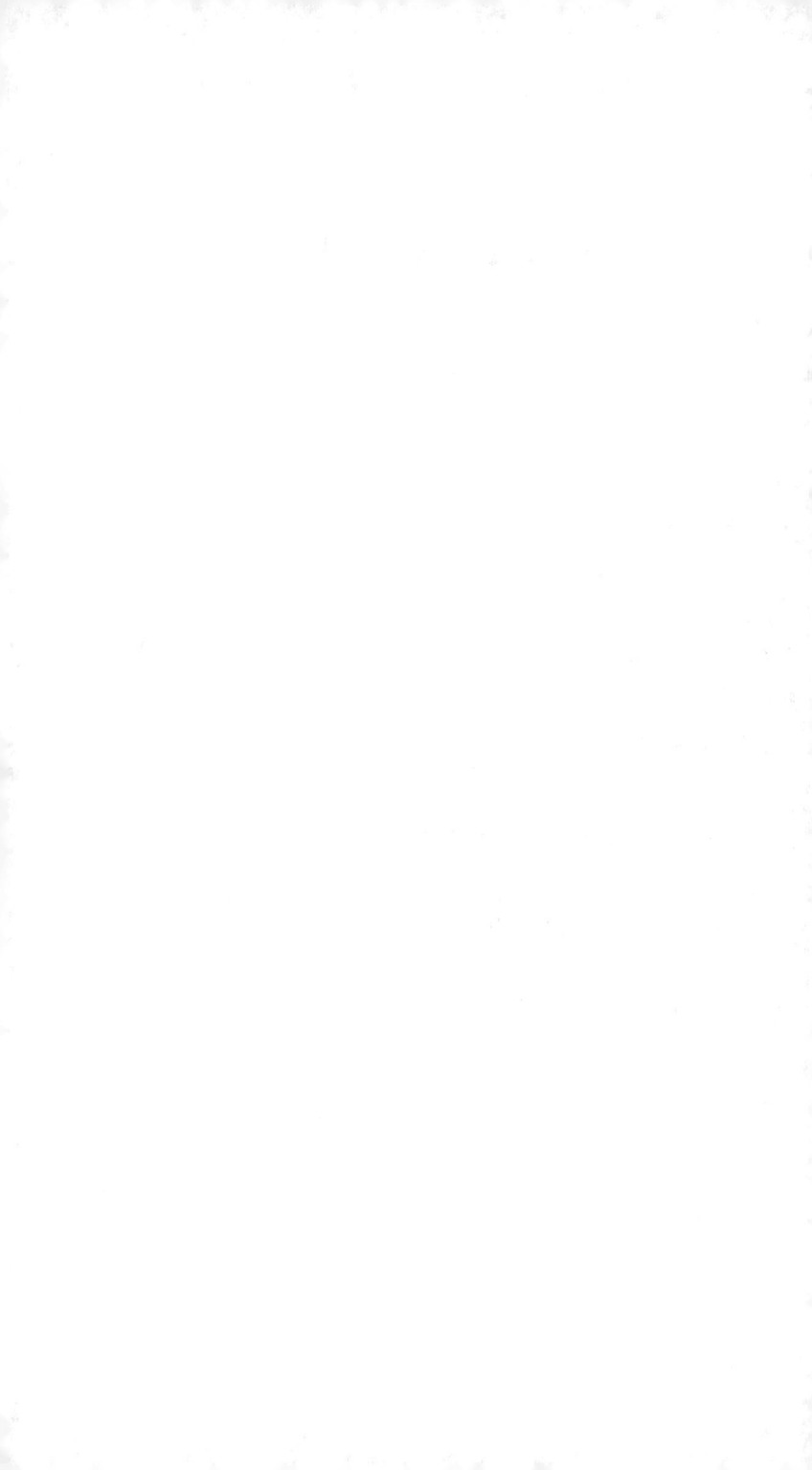

Introduction

Let me just say right now that I am no model, and that by no means do I have 100% flawless skin. I do, however, have 100% healthier, happier skin that I feel confident in. I believe that we all have the ability to be happy and healthy with skin that reflects the natural beauty we all possess.

In my twenties, I once had no hope that I could be blemish free. I felt doomed to hide beneath makeup every day for the rest of my life. In my searches for skin clarity, I had just about tried it all. I had chemical peels, microdermabrasion treatments, facials, IPL lasers, and used every acne product out there short of Accutane.

While some of those treatments seemed to momentarily help, there was never a product that gave noticeable, effective results. I was at war with my skin. I was losing the battle. I felt ugly.

I was mad that I had to deal with these embarrassing breakouts well past high school and that anger spilled into other areas of my life. I didn't want to leave the house or meet new people. I wasn't myself. I was miserable. Does that sound familiar?

I finally decided enough was enough. I knew I could have clear skin, I just had to figure out how. If other people did, so could I. This is probably the biggest secret to success I've discovered on my journey. I committed to changing the way I approached skin care.

After stepping back and having a deep look into my lifestyle and product usage, I was able to pick out the issues. I did some research. And some more research. Pretty soon I was all-consumed, spending weeks researching skincare until it finally clicked.

Everything made so much sense suddenly. I started seeing results that blew me away. I was excited by the progress I saw EVERY DAY. I knew I had to share these secrets with the world because I know how it feels to think you'll never be clear. That awful feeling doesn't have to last.

You CAN have clear skin, all you need to do is decide it's possible.

I want to applaud you for taking that first step to the best skin of your life. If I could, I'd jump up and down and give you a hug, that's how exciting this is! This book outlines the path to skin freedom.

If you can follow the advice in this book, you will see dramatic improvements in your skin's tone, texture, and overall clarity. The best part is: you will save hundreds, maybe thousands of dollars on skin care while becoming happier, healthier and freeing up so much time. If that's not a victory, I don't know what is!

Now that I've been through this cleanse and followed the tips I'm sharing with you here, I'm a woman happy in her skin, free from persistent acne, redness, and hypersensitivity. I no longer worry about spending those thirty (often more) minutes in front of the mirror every morning and night feeling stressed over the state of my complexion.

I don't need to wear foundation anymore. I can fall asleep without the dreaded time consuming routine most so-called experts advise. I wake up without fear that I will see a fresh crop of bumps on my face in the morning. I'm free from the chains of the skin care routine and I'm here to tell you: you can be too!

This is what has worked for me and countless other men and women. A simple anti-cleansing period of thirty days will help your skin rebuild the protective barrier that all those cleansers and products have stripped away. After thirty days you'll reveal new, healthier skin.

It will be tough to let go of the reigns, but if you can do it for thirty days, you won't ever look back. You'll jumpstart healing from the inside out and learn to listen to your body. The biggest hurdle most people have is allowing the body to do what it needs to do to heal. We want to "help the process along" by using these creams, scrubs and toners.

We're impatient. We want what we want when we want it. Unfortunately, this is just not a realistic approach when it comes to our health. The truth is: your skin has been pleading with you to back away and let it do its job. It's time to listen.

I finally listened to my body and I wish I would have done it years ago. Life is way too short to suffer with embarrassing acne and low self-esteem. It's time to stop punishing your skin with chemicals and feed it from the inside out so that it can become healthy, nourished and clear.

If you can be strong for thirty days and actively listen to your body, you WILL notice a difference. Are you ready?

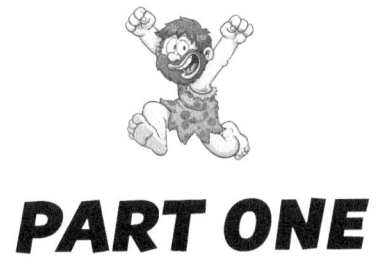

PART ONE

All About Your Skin

1

About This Cleanse

The Caveman Cleanse goes like this: Leave your face alone. Don't wash it, don't moisturize it, don't cover it in makeup. Don't touch it. Leave. It. Alone. Pretty simple, right? That's it. That's the basic philosophy behind having great skin.

If you think about it, our cavemen ancestors didn't wash their faces and it's safe to say they probably got dirtier than any of us have in our lifetime. I know what you're thinking, and yes, that was a long time ago. Humankind has come a long way technologically and intellectually speaking; but evolution-wise, in the last few hundred years, we haven't changed all that much genetically.

We are still pretty much the same creatures we were thousands of years ago. As the theory goes, it takes about one million years for any notable evolutionary changes to be seen. This means that our skin is still functioning the way it did long before soaps and cleansers were ever invented.

While I'm certainly not about to tell you to go live in a cave or club something (or someone) over the head, I do have to say *it makes a lot of sense that our skin should be able to take care of itself without our help.*

Since we are very adept creatures, it's only logical to trust our bodies to do their jobs.

It's unnatural to use a cleanser on your face. Skin simply wasn't designed for it. It was carefully engineered to take care of itself all on its own.

You see, our skin has an acid mantle which is a combination of dead skin cells, sweat, oil and good bacteria that act as a barrier to protect our body from external contaminants like makeup, artificial moisturizers, pollutants, you name it; this acid mantle is what keeps our complexion in balance.

Therefore, when we are consistently washing it away with cleansers and smothering it in moisturizers, we are getting rid of our skin's natural ability to care for itself.

This means irritation, breakouts, redness, flakiness, eczema, oiliness, and a host of other skin conditions. *Conditions which make the cosmetic industry money.*

They cause you these problems with the products they sell you, then they market another product that is supposed to fix the issue and you get trapped in a cycle of treatments, cleansers and routines that just plain don't do any good.

You think, "Wait a minute, you're telling me this layer of dead skin, oil and sweat are supposed to be there? Doesn't this go against everything we've ever been told?"

Yes!

Our bodies are these stellar machines that when allowed to do their jobs, are capable of amazing things and clear skin is part of that.

Your body knows what its doing and the Caveman Cleanse will help you realize that. It's not just about looking great on the outside. It's about feeling good inside, feeling healthy, sexy, strong, confident and just plain badass.

Once you learn to relinquish control over your skin, you will feel true freedom. You will stop buying into the cosmetic industry's claims to beautiful skin by way of the latest chemical-laden craze. You'll start to question what else you've always been told you need to do, only to find that's likely not the case; but that's a whole other matter worthy of its own book!

Imagine this: you spend your day however you feel and fall into bed without washing your face. How about getting an extra hour of sleep because you don't need to spend that time washing, toning, moisturizing and covering up your skin? Go camping without stressing about being able to do your lengthy skin care routine.

Get a little dirt on your face without the anxiety attack that you might now have a breakout brewing. Sleep over at someone's house without fearing they will see you without makeup or question what's taking you so long in the bathroom.

It's true freedom, and it's truly life-changing.

I began this Caveman Cleanse as a last resort, after a fit of "screw-it-nothing-works-anyway" depression. I figured, why waste time and money on all those stupid products that worked for the first few days and quit working soon after, leaving my skin red, irritated and worse than before?

I was at the lowest of lows when it comes to self-esteem. Twenty-two, working in the business world where appearance is as important as aptitude if you want to be taken seriously.

I felt nobody would take me seriously with a face full of acne. I wanted to look people in the eye with confidence that comes from knowing they aren't seeing all my imperfections the moment they meet me. Who doesn't want to feel confident in their skin?

So, I ditched all the products. I took the facial cleansers, masks, scrubs, and toners out of my bathroom and hid them from sight so I wouldn't cave in my moments of weakness when my need for control was at its strongest. I avoided the mirror as much as I could while my skin was healing. I got back into my hobbies and started crafting, writing and reading.

I did everything I could think of to keep from touching my face and obsessing over it in the mirror.

Strangely enough, nobody seemed to notice the difference. Nobody looked at me incredulously for not wearing makeup. Nobody said anything or stared. I expected some dramatic scene to break out, but nothing happened. I went about my business as usual and so did everybody else.

It's so very easy not to wash your face. Not moisturizing it is a total cake walk. Gloriously simple.

That's the beauty of it all: you simply have to do nothing.

Once you can get over the anxiety of quitting your products and adjusting to your new non-routine, you'll be amazed at how much your attitude will change, not to mention how much more time you'll have! You'll become happier and you'll take on a more spontaneous view of the world. Weekend road trips on a moment's notice? Sure. Ten minutes to throw some clothes and toothbrush in a bag and you are good to go. Freedom. Finally!

You ask: What if I work out and get sweaty? Rinse with water and gently pat your face dry. If you must wear mascara, remove it with coconut oil. You can warm it in your clean hands and gently apply the oil over your lashes, wipe clean with a wet cotton pad or washcloth, then rinse your face of any residue and pat dry. Bonus! This method works much better than store bought eye makeup remover, is much cheaper, and is conditioning for your skin and lashes. Avoid makeup as much as possible, you're going to be surprised at what you'll find in most cosmetics later in this book.

Now, I know what you're thinking: Don't wash my face? Are you crazy?! I'll be an oily, gross, dirty mess! No can do. No makeup? Not happening.

I'm telling you: the world will keep turning. You can do it. Especially if I did. It's worse in theory than it is in action. The scariest part is in your head.

I was the most product addicted person I know.

I had all kinds of toners, cleansers, masks, scrubs, moisturizers, serums, spot treatments and any other magic potion that promised smooth skin. And I used them all, sometimes at once. There would be days I'd wash then scrub, then use a mask, after that a toner, spot treatment, serum and moisturizer. Holy cow. The thought of doing that now makes me cringe.

If you think it'll be hard, I'm telling you now, the worst part is all in your head. I'll share with you my experience just as I journaled it in the first thirty days of the cleanse, emotions and all.

I urge you to do the same. Use this journal section to write it all down. As you look back, it will be easier to pick out the triggers and habits.

My experience the first thirty days:

Day 1

I showered and tried to keep my face out of the water this morning. Patted my face dry and didn't use a moisturizer.

There wasn't any oiliness or dryness. I wore a little mineral makeup to even out redness and angry looking spots. Rinsed my face gently with water at night.

Days 2 through 4

My face seemed to be noticeably more even toned. Nothing miraculous, but I noticed a difference from the typical redness I'd experience post-cleansing from getting out of the shower.

I still wetted my face when I showered and gently patted it dry. This helped me to fight the urge to use a cleanser. I found it hard to break the routine of cleansing and moisturizing and wearing makeup.

I didn't wear any makeup for these days. It was a test to my confidence. I felt nearly naked like everyone was looking at my skin, though it was really my own paranoia. Confidence wasn't at an all time high. I still couldn't stop touching my face, which I know contributed to some irritation. It was also difficult being without makeup.

Day 5

I noticed dryness around my chin and a little bit on my forehead. It was to the point that I wanted to scratch off the flakiness, and while I can't say that I behaved a 100%, what I did do was gently rub the flaky areas with clean fingers and if they didn't very easily lift away, I left them alone.

It was strange to me because after barely touching my face in the past I always noticed how red and irritated it would look immediately afterward, and it didn't seem to be the case today.

However, I reminded myself this is part of what caused the problem and that helped me to calm my bad habit of touching my face.

Day 7

The dryness has persisted. I've decided to hydrate more from the inside out and have upped my water intake. I've noticed a difference foremost in my lips. The more hydrated I am, the plumper my lips look.

Also, my skin looks less dull and better toned when I am properly hydrated. I've also been more diligent in taking my fish oil and evening primrose supplements. They seem to play a big role in the overall healthy look of my skin.

Day 9

I've been noticing flakey patches over some of the post-inflammatory marks on my face as well as the recently healing blemishes. It seems like my face is finally taking over its natural process and beginning to heal without all the interference from my "miracle" products.

My face is doing a better job of healing itself than that $30 cleanser and $28 moisturizer. Funny, isn't it, that letting go of your control and letting your body do what it was designed to do, yields better results than money can buy?

I didn't wear makeup today either. It's starting to not bother me so much. I'm getting used to seeing myself without makeup on and it's been an intriguing journey so far.

I've noticed more buildup of dry skin on my forehead, mostly because it's itchy as hell at times and I can't stand not being allowed to scratch it. The overall color and texture is better than it has ever been.

Day 10

I wore some concealer on the spots to help keep my spirits up through this healing process. The texture is noticeably better, I'd say about a 60% improvement from day one, and it hasn't even been two weeks. What skin care product can promise that and deliver?

I used to have small bumps on my chin called milia, which were essentially not acne, but buildup of skin cells and extra proteins that supposedly could only be removed by exfoliating on the regular. So not true. That exfoliation seemed to be causing the problem.

The more products I used, the worse my face had become. The more I let go, the better. Ironic isn't it? I have no more milia bumps!

By now, the pimples that I do get come and go almost before I even notice them and they aren't the crazy, red, angry looking things that used to torment me before. They are those ones that you see those crazy models on tv pretending to stress over. As in, they blend in with my skin tone and you don't see them unless you are two inches from my face, which you aren't. So I don't even stress them, I leave them alone, and then they disappear. I can deal with those on occasion.

My skin tone looks better every day. Again, the dry skin is noticeable if I scratch my forehead more than gently.

I've started changing up my diet a little bit, trying to align more closely to the raw, unpackaged, unprocessed wholesome food of my caveman ancestors.

I've incorporated more fish oil supplements, because I still can't bring myself to pretend I love the taste of fish(call me crazy, I know). The supplements are working famously, so I will keep at it. I like what those omegas do for my skin. I've still been guzzling the water = amazing for the body and mind.

I'm not drinking any dairy, including lattes. I'm a little sad about that, but I'll get over it. I've been in the habit of eating two eggs for breakfast in the morning, trying to get back to basics and stay away from packaged foods as much as humanly possible.

It's crazy how much more energy I've had over the past few days. I've noticed that evening primrose oil has been a tremendous helper in regulating my hormonal mood swings and monthly breakouts. I've been taking that for a few months now and have noticed improvement, but when combined with this new regimen of not using cleansers, moisturizers or makeup, it's shown me the power of hormones.

I'm cutting back on sugar and finding new ways to keep my mind occupied rather than spending time in front of the mirror stressing over my skin. I've taken up meditation which has been a life saver in calming me down when I feel stressed out.

Day 11
I left on the little spots of makeup I put on yesterday. Woke up. Crazy thing happened: the world kept turning and my face didn't explode like Vesuvius. Had a few flakey patches that I've come to accept

as healing these days. It is appreciative and has rewarded my self-confidence with no redness or irritation. It's still healing. I'm happier letting it do its thing and not stressing about which product I have to use which time of day and which day of the week.

This has been the part where I'm learning to de-stress. I've been getting more sleep at night since I don't have to spend 30 minutes cleansing and obsessing before bed. I fall into bed after brushing my teeth not worrying about what happens if I don't wash my face.

I wake up in the morning, half an hour later than usual, and I don't stress it, because I wake up ready. As mother nature intended.

I've forced myself to step back from the mirror, stop leaning in closer over the counter to dissect my imperfections and think: people see me from this distance. Nobody is going to be as close to my face as this mirror I'm deathly close to right now, so why I am stressing about something nobody else will notice? Furthermore, who the heck cares?!

Since I've stopped washing and doing really anything to my face except for the occasional splash of water and mascara removal with coconut oil, it's become incredibly obvious the repercussions of my diet on my skin. I now know what in my diet is causing me to break out since I've eliminated all other irritants. I see what makes my skin seem to glow. I have better control of what I put into my body because I'm putting nothing on my skin.

Day 13

I went out shopping with a friend. Listened to a skincare saleswoman do her pitch on why this brand was amazing and why she needed to cleanse and tone and moisturize on top of exfoliating and using a mask four days out of the week.

I heard her talk, but I couldn't help but notice that her face didn't look any better than mine did before I started this cleanse 13 days ago. In fact, it looked almost worse than mine does now.

So as I'm listening to her telling me how these products have helped her face tremendously after listing off the overwhelming amount of products she used, I again study her skin and I notice something: that "brightening" eye cream doesn't make her eyes look any more shimmery or light than the next person. That clay mask didn't clear anything up worth mentioning.

When I get to thinking about it again… I can't bring myself to break my cleanse to try these miracle products. I think, maybe at the thirty day mark I will try a little bit of the "all natural" gentle exfoliating scrub, and maybe a clay mask. But maybe not. I will listen to what my skin needs.

The biggest thing I've learned so far is to listen to my body and trust it. All the problems I feel like

I've ever had have come from not listening to that voice and allowing myself to be misguided by the weird stigmas just like those that tell us we must wash our faces twice a day.

That should be a huge red flag! **What could I possibly be doing that warrants me to wash off that protective barrier twice a day?** I'm not slathering my face with a bunch of gunk or rolling around in something sticky, so why do I need to wash it twice a day with some harsh chemical-laden creation that was conjured in some lab somewhere with who-knows-what-that-ingredient-is-because-I-can't-pronounce-it!?

Let go and let Mother Nature take the reins. She knows what she's doing. She's been doing it much longer than you have.

Day 15

My face still seems to be in the healing phase. I had a few nondescript new blemishes. They were gone pretty much the day they appeared. My chin still has a few healing breakouts from "that time of the month" and my boyfriend refusing to shave.

I don't seem to wake up to overly flakey skin anymore. The texture on my forehead and nose is feeling a bit rough like really fine grit sandpaper, though it seems less easily irritated than it ever has been.

I'm still seeing a few patches of dead skin on my

chin and around my mouth on the post-acne marks and I'm thinking those spots have begun to get lighter, though it could be my imagination or wishful thinking.

I very lightly and gently exfoliated with a washcloth more to ease my anxiety than for any other reason. It helped alleviate some of the stress I felt about not having control over my skin, while allowing me a little "cheat" without totally breaking the rules.

I feel that not stressing out is the biggest factor in skin care and overall health. Happy people are the prettiest people, after all. That and learning to keep my damn hands off my face. Once I can stop that compulsion, I think I will be in the clear.

Day 29
I've noticed improvement in my hyperpigmentation marks. They are still getting flaky on top and lightening. I think this will continue if I keep up my simple regimen and clean up my diet. It's been nice to stop sitting around obsessing about my face.

Day 32
I went out with my man last night and wore a little makeup on the spots and swiped on some mascara. I didn't wash any of it off before I went to bed and woke up in the morning with a new breakout in the area I applied the makeup.

This lead me to believe my makeup was partly to

blame for my skin woes. I researched the ingredients in my makeup. My eyes have never been so big! I couldn't believe companies are allowed to put that stuff in cosmetics! No freaking wonder my face was so irritated before. I returned all the makeup I could gather receipts for.

Day 35

I gently and lightly exfoliated the layer of dead skin using a sample of the Origins Modern Friction exfoliating product and I almost wish I hadn't, simply because my skin looked irritated for the rest of the night. I had grown used to my more dull-but-not red-and-therefore-better-looking face.

After pouting for the night, I took my milk thistle, evening primrose and fish oil supplements with my vitamin and went to bed. I awoke to skin that appeared more even and much softer than it had all month. It wasn't dry or oily at all, and it wasn't covered in a thicker than normal layer of dead skin.

Since I've quit touching my face, I've noticed a HUGE decrease in the number of breakouts I get each month.

I'm still working on getting my hormones and sugar consumption under control, but all in all, I can tell that I'm making progress because the severity and number of breakouts have dramatically decreased.

2

How Your Skin Works

By now, it's probably not news that your skin is the largest organ of the body; but did you know that all 22 square feet of skin that make up the average adult are responsible for signaling to the immune system an impending attack from germs? Your skin is what helps regulate your body temperature, ensuring you maintain a nice and toasty average of 98 degrees.

Maybe you were unaware that the skin is made up of three layers: the dermis, the epidermis, and the subcutis. You see, aside from physically holding you together, your skin is an amazing organ that has more jobs than your average factory. Let's take a look at each of the layers in a little more depth.

At the very bottom of your skin is the base layer, also known as the subcutis or hypodermis. The subcutis is a network of loose connective tissue and an insulating layer of fat that acts as a fuel reserve in the event of a food shortage. It insulates your innards from knocks and falls and is the foundation that all other layers rest atop.

Just above the hypodermis sits the dermis which is made up of collagen and elastin, fibers that help to give your skin its strength and elasticity.

The blood vessels in this layer of skin are smaller than those in the hypodermis. They help regulate your body temperature by expanding to allow heat to escape and restricting the blood flow when it's cold. Pain, temperature, and touch are all sensed by a vast network of nerves contained here that carry messages to brain.

This is also the level at which your hair follicles and glands with ducts (AKA your pores) begin. The Apocrine glands, which develop during puberty, produce scented sweat linked to sexual attraction, which can cause that unpleasant body odor we have all had the displeasure of sniffing. Though it can be smelly (depending on your diet), sweat is entirely necessary to bring down the internal body temperature and rid the body of waste fluids.

Those sebacious glands we hear so much about are responsible for secreting oil-like sebum that keeps our skin and hair moisturized and healthy. This layer is the workhorse when it comes to keeping the body in balance.

Working our way outward, we come to the layer bonded on top of the dermis: the epidermis. This is the outermost layer of skin. It's mostly made of keratinocytes. These little buggers are the cells on the outer surface of the epidermis.

The very top layer is composed of dead skin that forms a tough protective layer allowing new cells underneath to continuously regenerate and make their way to the surface.

Keratin is that awesome protein that helps give our skin, hair, and nails their strength. These keratino-cytes make up many tiny cells that are constantly expanding and growing outwards as the surface cells die and flake off.

It takes about five weeks for newly created cells to work their way to the surface. This layer of dead skin is known as the stratum corneum and just above it is the acid mantle. The stratum corneum varies in thickness throughout the body (think of the difference between the soles of your feet and the skin around your eyes).

In this acid mantle are one of the body's many defense mechanisms: Langerhans cells. These bad boys are what let your immune system know viruses and other infectious agents are on the prowl. There's also a microscopic ecosystem of good bacteria in the acid mantle made of secretions from sweat, oil, and lipids.

The acid mantle is home to enzymes that help break down sebum to prevent it from clogging inside the pores. It maintains that balance of sebum so skin stays moisturized and supple and prevents it from cracking and becoming damaged or infected. These helpful bacteria boost the immune system so it can produce antigens close to the surface of the skin that retard the growth of pathogens and bad bacteria.

With all the environmental stressors like exhaust fumes, pollutants, UV rays, dust, makeup, cleansers, toners, moisturizers, even air conditioning, our skin works over time to protect us from inflammation, skin damage and sensitivity.

On their own, the aforementioned toxins can break down our natural defense mechanisms and interrupt the functions of the epidermis. Once this happens, our skin gets knocked out of balance and bacteria find the secret passage ways through the stratus corneum just below.

This is where our acid mantle comes to the rescue. If it hasn't been washed away by harsh cleansers and astringents, this protective barrier helps fight off invaders, keeping in moisture that makes our skin look and feel soft and smooth and protects it from becoming sensitized or irritated.

This skin "fortress" is strengthened by skin cells, proteins, oils, and lipids. This system of bricks and mortar retain the water that is essential to healthy skin function. If we focus on the acid mantle for a moment longer, it's easy to see why it's so important to be aware of what you put on your skin. If it ever feels irritated or inflamed, the barrier function is probably impaired.

To treat the many skin issues such as acne, dryness, irritation, oiliness, and sensitivity, we need to look under the surface to be sure we aren't inadvertently harming our skin. By washing away the acid mantle, essentially, the skin is peeled open to allow harmful bacteria and pollution to cause further damage.

Keep this barrier intact and quit waging a war on it with unnatural products. You deserve to have healthy skin!

3

Are You Causing Your Acne?

Are you one of those people who spend a lot of time in front of the mirror examining your pores, trying out the newest cleansers, toners, and scrubs? Do you switch makeups and concealers often, hoping to find one that won't make you break out?

Have you spent countless hours perusing the beauty aisles, comparing products? Do you scrub your face at least every other day, maybe every day? Does your bathroom counter rival your favorite beauty supply store? If any of this sounds familiar, you may be causing your acne.

I'm so glad it finally dawned on me that I was causing myself the majority of my skin issues. I could not stop touching my face. I saw a pimple- I had to pop it, therefore creating more redness and acne in the process. And then more popping, resulting in a lot of acne and lot of stress and a lot of touching my face to feel the new bumps I had caused. It's a bad habit that I learned the consequences of the hard way.

If you pick at your face, you will get scars. As if the acne itself isn't bad enough, you get to be reminded on a daily basis that you used to have a horrible acne problem.

Don't pick your face! It will heal exponentially slower if you do. And it will be angrier looking while it does! Don't do it. Not even once.

In an effort to be rid of those bumps, you scrub and scrub, and cleanse and spot "treat" and tone and moisturize, and otherwise punish your skin in an effort to control its behavior.

The desperate need for control is the heart of many acne problems. It's HUGE. While you mean well and at the time feel like you are doing something good for your skin, you still go to sleep with redness and wake up with new zits.

Then you think: I didn't clean that area well enough, or I didn't use enough salicylic acid or benzoyl peroxide. Or maybe your skin is dry and you think, I didn't apply enough moisturizer or I didn't exfoliate well enough. *That's what we've been trained to think. That's what makes companies money and makes you breakout.* And I'm here to tell you, it's wrong! So very wrong.

Here are a few indicators you are causing your breakouts:

- You touch your face. Even without realizing it sometimes, you rest your chin in your hand. Or you get stressed and rub your forehead. Maybe you do the thinking man pose with your fingers stroking your chin thoughtfully. Strange, that's where you see the most pimples…

- Your phone is pressed up against your face as you're talking, after your fingers have been swiping the screen all day. It hides at the bottom of your purse, along with your keys that get dropped on the ground, or your makeup bag that never gets washed. It's probably fallen onto the floor of your car at least a time or two.

You would never put your face anywhere you put your phone, yet there it is on your cheek where you see quite a few breakouts.

- You love the cold side of the pillowcase. So you flip your pillow over. And over. Maybe you drool a little bit. Wait, when was the last time you washed that thing or swapped it out for a fresh one? Change your pillowcase often. I have accumulated a collection of pillowcases so I can swap them out every other day without having to do a bunch of laundry. It's a small price to pay for beautiful skin. Besides, who doesn't love a fresh clean pillowcase?

- Your hair, it looks amazing. It sure didn't get that way without gel, mousse, hair spray, or serum. It falls flat against your forehead and you find your forehead feeling a little greasy. Or maybe its long and swaying in the breeze and against your jaw, or getting caught on your lip gloss. You pull it away inadvertently sliding it across your face, styling products and all. Keep your hair off your face as much as possible

That detergent you bought because it smells amazing. Newsflash: it takes a whole lot of fragrance and chemicals to make it smell that way, and not a one of those are skin-friendly.

- Ladies: Does your man have an epic beard or a funky 'stache? Yes, that facial hair may be glorious, but all those prickly man-hairs rubbing against your face aren't doing your skin any favors. Hello, irritation!

You drink soda when you should be drinking water. This doesn't need to be explained. Drink more water.

- You sleep with your long hair loose and wild. Tie it up at night. All those beautiful oils are good for your scalp and hair, but they don't belong on your face and neither do your hair products.
- Do you shampoo and condition before or after you rinse your face? Those lingering amounts of conditioner and shampoo can sit on your

skin, overloading it with foreign oils and waxes. Rinse your face well after rinsing your hair.

Have your friends never seen you without your favorite baseball hat? And the pimples on your forehead beneath it? Hats get dirty, and they don't get washed often, if ever. Try giving your skin a break for a while, see what happens.

- Those teeth need to stay clean and bright, so I'm not about to tell you to ditch your toothpaste. However, be aware of where the toothpaste ends up. If you're seeing a rise in bumps around your mouth, your toothpaste may be to blame.

Fluoride, while it gets mixed reviews about doing more harm than good, is almost certainly a contributor to mouth area breakouts as it is an irritant and often comes into contact with that area of the face. Try keeping the toothpaste in your mouth as much as possible to avoid contact with your skin and rinse your chin and mouth area after brushing and flossing. Opt for a fluoride-free natural alternative toothpaste.

- Do you eat spicy or greasy foods and slurp your soup and pasta? All that slurping and burger-noshing could be to blame for breakouts on your chin, cheeks and around your mouth. Rinse the food off your face after you've fed it.

Chores won't do themselves, true, but if you're

constantly exposed to harsh chemicals like bleach or kitchen cleaner, you could be exposing yourself to many more toxins than you realize. You clean the bathtub and suddenly your face itches, or your back itches and of course, you have to scratch it. In desperate need for relief, you skip the hand washing and scratch the itch, with all those cleaners and germs under your nails and all over your fingers.

Are you heavy handed with your washcloth? Never, ever rub your face with a towel, pat it dry very gently.

Stop stressing so much! You've heard it a thousand times. And I'm telling you for the thousandth and one time: chill out. There are things outside your control sometimes.

Take a deep breath. A nifty breathing trick that I actually use: Breathe in for ten slow seconds, hold it for ten slow seconds and exhale for ten more slow seconds. Visualize something that makes you happy: a puppy, a giggly baby, sand beneath your toes. You know what it is. Think about it and breathe. Observe your emotions without attaching to them. Repeat until the stress subsides. It's gloriously simple.

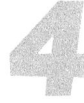

Let Your Skin Breathe

Your skin needs oxygen just as much as your lungs do. It needs oxygen to repair itself from free radical damage and oxidation. Just like a wound needs air to heal, so does skin. It helps to keep the balance. All those products you're using are smothering your skin and confusing it. You're inadvertently sabotaging the health of your skin.

Quit the salicylic acid and the benzoyl peroxide.

You wouldn't intentionally burn yourself, would you? Well, that's what those products do. Stop putting ACID on your face. It's not natural and it's not healthy. You'll be shocked to learn what's in some of those things we use on a daily basis.

Let's start with benzoyl peroxide. The CDC classifies benzoyl peroxide as a combustible solid, easily ignited and it burns very rapidly. It's extremely explosion sensitive to shock, heat and friction, as well as heat and static discharge. The Material Safety Data Sheet on the chemical benzoyl peroxide lists it as *"very hazardous in case of skin contact"* and instructs, *"in case of contact, flush thoroughly with water, disinfect and cover with antibiotic cream; seek medical attention immediately."*

It also says to keep away from direct sunlight. It doesn't seem possible to escape the sun these days and it seems to me all those risks are really not worth it. It's a nasty irritant that causes redness and peeling. I don't know about you, but the last thing I want to do is make my already noticeable pimple glowing red and flakey looking.

What about salicylic acid you say? Glad you asked. It's even worse, and it seems to be in every single acne product out there. Notice they are called "acne products", because that's what they do: cause acne.

Hydroxybenzoic acid, AKA salicylic acid, contains carbon dioxide, an oxidative substance which prematurely ages the skin.

It penetrates skin cells to cause damage and slows the ability of skin to heal itself. This is exactly the opposite effect we are looking for when we think of clearing our acne. Yet, this light and moisture-sensitive chemical makes its way into makeup bags and medicine cabinets everywhere.

The Material Safety Data Sheet on salicylic acid

lists it as *"Hazardous in case of skin contact, of eye contact, and of inhalation. Causes dermatitis. Severe over exposure can result in death. It is a developmental toxin and highly toxic to the reproductive systems. Repeated exposure to a highly toxic material may produce general deterioration of health by an accumulation in one or many human organs. Seek medical attention in case of skin contact. It's not to be stored above 73.4 degrees fahrenheit."*

There aren't many people who aren't exposed to temperatures above 74 degrees for at least part of the year. It's unstable in excessive heat (think summertime pretty much anywhere) and dust and is incompatible with moisture. Let's hope your face never gets wet.

Oh, and it's reactive to light. Better stay in a cave in middle earth somewhere if you want to use this stuff with a lowered risk of spontaneous combustion! (Okay, yes, that may be a little dramatic, but I need to stress just how awful this stuff really is).

According to the Data Sheet *"Salicylic acid may affect genetic material. It is transferred into breast milk and is embryo-toxic, meaning harmful to a developing baby. It affects the cardiovascular system, increasing blood pressure and body temperature.*

It causes coughing, difficulty breathing, ringing in the ears, confusion, rapid heart rate, headache, dizziness, nausea, vomiting, possible kidney damage, and depression. Prolonged exposure may cause dermatitis. Affects the central nervous system and the acid-base balance in the body, resulting in delirium and tremors". And this ingredient is everywhere! EEK!

These are all things the cosmetic industry won't tell you. It's poison. Plain and simple. As if the feeling of seeing your acne in the mirror wasn't disheartening on its own, you're slathering on a chemical that has been proven to cause depression, birth defects, delirium and a host of other nasty things.

Let's talk about other products that you may be using on your body. Think of a very well-known baby shampoo and baby oil company. These products contain ingredients such as dioxane, quaternium 15, and mineral oil, proven cancer causing ingredients.

"Dioxane forms explosive peroxides, causes respiratory, eye, and skin irritation. It's listed as a possible cancer hazard. Its targeted organs are: kidneys, central nervous system, liver, respiratory system, eyes, and skin.

It causes skin irritation. May be harmful if absorbed through the skin. Repeated or prolonged exposure may cause drying and cracking of the skin. May cause irritation of the digestive tract. May cause central nervous system depression, characterized by excitement, followed by headache, dizziness, drowsiness, and nausea.

Advanced stages may cause collapse, unconscious-ness, coma and possible death due to respiratory failure.

May be harmful if swallowed. Inhalation of high con-centrations may cause central nervous system effects characterized by nausea, headache, dizziness, un-consciousness and coma. Causes respiratory tract irritation. May cause liver and kidney damage.

Possible cancer hazard based on tests with laboratory animals. Adverse reproductive effects have been reported in animals. Laboratory experiments have resulted in mutagenic effects. Chronic exposure may cause blood effects. Animal studies have reported the development of tumors."

Quaternium -15 releases the preservative formal-dehyde, an embalming fluid. Severe over exposure can result in death.

Mineral oil, formed from the distillation of petroleum, was shown to increase tumor growth 69% in an animal study. It causes estrogen dominance as it is a xenoestrogen. It suffocates the skin and hinders all rejuvenation.

Cosmetics are just as bad. Many of them contain dimethicone, propylene glycol, ascorbyl palmitate, tocopheryl, parabens, the list goes on and on. These and many other ingredients in cosmetics are known cancer causing ingredients.

It's best to avoid makeup if possible. If you simply

can't be without it, do your research and look at the ingredient labels, be suspicious of long lists and anything you can't easily pronounce. Use only natural ingredients. It'll take more effort, but your health is certainly worth it.

I wouldn't knowingly put myself or a child anywhere near chemicals like that, in any concentration, yet they are found in baby products, body washes, cosmetics, and the like. **Be aware of what you are buying!** Do your research! I cannot urge this strongly enough.

Rather than punishing your skin with these products time and again, give it a breather and let it heal from the inside out. Nourish it so that it can heal and glow.

Earth has given us all we need to be healthy. There are so many alternatives out there to use in place of commercial products. It simply takes a little research and trial to see what your body responds to best.

Healthy Alternatives to Everyday Products

Moisturizers:
- Jojoba oil
- Olive oil
- Raw shea butter

Exfoliants:
- Fresh lemon juice
- Baking soda
- Brown sugar

Cleansers:
- Water
- Castille soap
- Active Manuka Honey (rated 15+ UMF, OMA or 250+ MGO from New Zealand where the Manuka bush is native)
- Plain whole fat yogurt
- Olive, coconut, and jojoba oil

Masks:
Be careful not to let them dry and use the right mask for your skin type.

- Oily skin: green, bentonite, and kaolin clays
- Sensitive: red or white clay
- Dry: red clay
- Dull tired skin: pink clay
- Orris root powder and water
- Chickpea flour and water for oily skin
- Baking soda and water

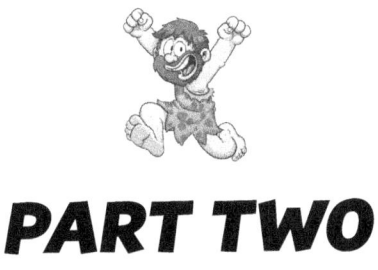

PART TWO

Heal Your Acne for Good,
the Holistic Way

5

Examine Your Diet
and Lifestyle

What does your day look like from start to finish? Do you wake up feeling stressed about the day ahead of you? Or are you excited for what's in store today? If your answer isn't the latter most days, I'm here to tell you, it should be. And it can be.

When you wake up in the morning, try to do something you don't normally do. For instance, if the first thing you do when you wake up is head for the bathroom, instead head for the kitchen and pour yourself a big glass of water. As you drink your water, think of a few things you want to accomplish for the day, visualize them happening and put on a smile.

Make small changes every day until you find the things you're doing are making you smile. For me, getting up in the morning and hitting the mat for a few sun salutations does the trick. I have a long commute most days, so I make sure to get pumped up by blasting some upbeat tunes and singing (quite horribly) to myself, so badly sometimes that I have to laugh at how tone deaf I am. This helps me feel at ease and remember to not take myself so seriously and have fun. The less stress I have, the better I feel and the better I look.

It's no secret acne can be caused by stress, so why not do what you can to minimize the daily stress? Do what you need to do to get happy. When you are happy, you feel good, you feel healthy, you have an aura about you that attracts the goodness you feel, and it's contagious to those around you. If your job is so stressful that you feel drained and burnt out, see if it's your perspective causing you to feel that way.

You can change your life by changing your perspective. If it's not the perspective that's off (as in, you no longer want to clean up the messes other people make or cook their food, or take orders from that soulless creature known as your boss), change the situation. Go back to school. Get that degree. Change careers. Do what you need to do to be happy.

Make happiness a priority every day.

Get moving. Our bodies were made to move, not to sit all day in front of a screen. You need to challenge your heart, get your blood pumping, get that oxygen into your skin. Go for a walk. Hike. Dance.

Run. Do something. Exercise is yet another way to rid your body of the toxins that may otherwise come out through your skin.

Its fun to let loose, don't get me wrong, but overdoing it often will have adverse effects on your skin and the rest of your body. If you find that you go out every Friday night for more than a few drinks, try cutting back a little. Alcohol dehydrates and does no favors for your skin or your liver (which is also crucial to keep healthy if you want great skin).

Think about what you are putting in your body. Do you regularly consume the items listed below?

Foods to Avoid:
- Fast food of any kind
- Microwave popcorn
- Soda
- High fructose corn syrup
- Soy milk
- Dairy (including cheese and yogurt)
- Chocolate
- Processed foods
- Foods with added sugar
- Packaged foods (mac and cheese, ramen noodle soup, chips, canned soup to name a few)
- White bread
- Trans fats

My Top Three Easy Glowing Skin Recipes:

Homemade pico de gallo salsa:

- 1 onion, finely chopped
- 1 medium tomato, diced
- 1/2 fresh jalapeno pepper, seeded and chopped
- 2 sprigs fresh cilantro, finely chopped
- 1 green onion, finely chopped
- 1 teaspoon finely chopped garlic
- Splash white vinegar
- 1/8 teaspoon pepper
- Fresh lime juice to taste

In a medium bowl, combine tomato, onion, jalapeno pepper, cilantro, and green onion. Season with fniely chopped garlic, lime and pepper. Mix well. Refrigerate for 30 minutes before eating.

Antioxidant berry banana super smoothie:

- strawberries
- blueberries
- raspberries
- one banana
- spinach
- almond milk

These recipes are very informal in nature. Play around with the ratios of fruit. I blend a handful of blueberries, about 7 strawberries and a banana with some spinach for good measure. Add un-sweetened vanilla almond milk as needed to blend. Frozen fruit is best for smoothies to keep the consistency smooth and creamy.

Green tea with lemon and raw honey:

Cut up a slice of lemon, squeeze and add it to hot water with a quarter size squirt of honey. Stir and add your tea bag or strainer. In addition to being great for the metabolism, this is also great for the immune system and ultra soothing for sore throats and sniffles.

Oatmeal with peanut butter, bananas, brown sugar and cinnamon:

Prepare whole grain oats as directed and add a heaping spoonful of peanut butter, a pinch of brown sugar and cinnamon sprinkled to taste. Cut up half a banana and add it in.Try adding slivered almonds for extra omegas and bit of a crunch.

Skin loving foods:

All fruits, especially lemons, grapefruits, oranges, limes, pomegranates, tomatoes, blueberries, strawberries and raspberries

All veggies, especially carrots, spinach, kale, bell peppers, and onions

Nuts: Almonds, sunflower seeds, and walnuts

Omegas: Peanut butter, salmon, quinoa

6

Learning to Listen to Your Body

This might be the toughest obstacle for many people. I know it was for me. Now, what exactly does it mean to listen to your body? It means that you pay attention to how the foods you eat affect your body. It means you get up and move when you feel restless, or you chill out when you're exhausted.

Ask yourself right now, "How do I feel?"

Do you feel good after you eat a high protein meal with veggies? Do you feel jittery after that cup of coffee? Did that burger just not sit well? For some reason, your skin suddenly looks better after you've had a big glass of water and a piece of fruit.

Maybe after a night of partying a little too hard and eating one too many fries or nachos, you waking up not looking or feeling so hot. A big deadline is leaving you feeling frayed and you just can't seem to concentrate anymore.

Your body clues you in about how it's doing, and while it may not be possible to head off every negative thing that comes your way, there are steps you can take to minimize the not so great effects on your body.

When choosing a certain behavior, ask your body, "How do feel about this?" And listen to it. You'll never regret listening to your gut. If your body sends out a sign of emotional or physical distress, think twice. If your body reacts with a signal of eagerness or comfort, go for it.

Your body is really good at telling you what it wants- it gives you plenty of clues. You'll feel it and you'll see it, if you know what to look for.

For instance, if you wash your face with a harsh cleanser, wash or scrub too vigorously, it looks red for anywhere from a few minutes to a few hours. Ever wonder why that is? You're irritating your skin. It's telling you the cleanser you're using isn't right for your skin, that it has something in it causing your skin damage, or that you are being too rough with your washing method.

You should never press hard into your skin to scrub it clean. This action creates micro-tears that are more easily inflamed and vulnerable to invading bacteria.

Mainstream cleansers like Clean and Clear, Neutrogena, and a good number of products work by sudsing away that protective acid mantle your skin needs to be healthy, to regulate its production of oils, fight off harmful bacteria, and heal itself.

You know that feeling you get after you wash your face, where your skin is tight enough to be mistaken for the head of a drum? Yeah, that's not normal. Your cleanser is taking away the good oils, which by the way, causes your skin to produce more and they tend to get trapped under all that synthetic moisturizer and makeup, leading to congestion that has nowhere to go but out. And you wake up with a new zit.

This is a great example of learning to listen to your body. Your skin shouldn't feel tight or be red after washing it. Those are signs that you're damaging your skin and causing it to age prematurely. Nobody wants that. Be gentle to your skin. Don't put anything on your skin that you wouldn't put in your mouth.

Remember that your mind and your body are holistic. Everything is connected. When one thing is out of balance, your body will tell you. When you learn to find balance, your body and mind will be at peace.

You cannot have a feeling, a sensation, or even a thought without the body. Always be listening to your body. Be constantly aware of yourself in your surroundings.

The power of awareness is what propels you upward. It is what connects your mind and body to each other. When you ignore the voice that whispers in your ear, you go against the flow of life, of nature. It's telling you what you need to do to keep the balance. When you listen to that voice, things seem to "go right" and you feel happy. When you ignore it, you get anxious, sad, or angry and your health is generally in a lowered state. These feelings and symptoms are signs that something is not right.

You need to take time every day to love yourself and take care of your whole self. You will radiate the health you are cultivating. Your skin will become clearer. Your mind will become clearer. You will be happier. You will make better choices and you will feed off the energy you generate through your awareness. You will reach new heights and this path to clear skin and happiness will catapult you to places you never knew existed. If you remember to remain aware, you will never run out of the fuel you need.

It's easy to get off track in your daily life; and it's just as easy to get back on. Take some time for yourself and do the things that bring your mind and body peace.

Meditate for a few minutes whenever you get the chance. This helps you to refocus and regain awareness and reconnect your mind and body. A good practice when meditating is to simply let thoughts come and go as they will. Do not attach yourself to your thoughts and feelings. Rather, observe them and let them run their course. You're teaching yourself to cope with stress and change your perspective and better your responses without even realizing it. This is a very powerful tool for becoming calm and centered.

Take a few moments to write about how you feel. When you feel happy, describe the way your day has gone and where the good energy comes from. When you're sad or angry, do the same. Writing about things that provoke emotions and sensations help you to see patterns and help you to become aware of the moments the tides begin to shift. You can change your sails before you get swept away into the storm if you learn to read the waters and the skies.

Understanding How Breakouts are Linked to Internal Health

Let's talk about hormones for a moment. Here's what you need to know: If you're a woman, your monthly dose of hormone-craziness can be controlled. If you're a man: it may be more difficult to spot a hormonal imbalance, but it is certainly doable.

We all need to balance our hormone levels and

there is no one-size-fits-all approach because only YOU know YOUR body. This is a massive component in the health of your skin. Since hormones control just about every process in the body from mood to digestion and energy levels, we need to learn to keep them under control. External hormones are BAD. Your body has all the hormones it needs, compliments of mother nature herself. The key to clear skin is balance.

I never used to understand what a tremendous role my hormones played in the clarity and overall quality of my skin. I also never understood what caused my hormones to be so out of whack.

After I began this Caveman Cleanse, I started to notice the correlation between the time of the month and the state of my complexion (and my sanity). After I learned to listen to my body I learned how to control and reduce monthly breakouts, mostly by observing cause and effect and writing down patterns I've noticed.

[Use this section to make notes of patterns you notice in your skin throughout the month, including diet and exercise.]

How to spot a hormonal imbalance:
1. You're constantly tired.
2. You're gaining weight and your diet isn't to blame.
3. You have wild mood swings.

4. You are forgetful and can't seem to focus.
5. You can't seem to get to sleep, or stay asleep.
6. You're never in "the mood".
7. Depression. Got a bad case of the blues?
8. You have achy joints.
9. Impaired immune system.
10. You guessed it- ACNE.

As a woman, your skin likely varies from week to week. Week one being the start of your period when your skin probably feels a little more sensitive, with new breakouts apparent.

Then comes week two, your body prepares for ovulation and your skin looks more even toned and is healing more rapidly.

By the middle of week two or maybe into week three (after all, every woman is different) you're ovulating at the very beginning of the week or you already have and you feel pretty. Your skin looks better, more even, less red and at the risk of being cliché, dare I say? glowing.

If you haven't become pregnant, your body sheds the unfertilized egg and uterine lining and prepares for menstruation. Week four: this is usually the peak of symptoms. Your body is more sensitive to pain and touch. Hello sore boobs and growling at your man for buying the vanilla ice cream instead of vanilla bean ice cream, because, hello! there's a huge difference! You just HAVE TO HAVE sugar, or salty foods, or maybe even a good cry. This is also when you get those painful, red bumps that seem to have set up camp on your face, usually along the jawline or around the mouth.

The reason these symptoms can be so severe is that you may have a hormone imbalance. It's not just women. Men may also have similar symptoms like anxiety, anger, sadness, and/or fatigue. While it's normal to experience these things once in a while, if you notice it on a regular basis, it's time to take a look at your hormones.

Androgens, the male hormones that are present in both men and women, can cause acne breakouts by altering the way skin cells in hair follicles develop in addition to over-stimulating oil glands.

All this extra oil gets trapped in the follicle and acne bacteria develops. The excess oil builds up and with nowhere else to go it erupts as a big fat zit. This is where the research usually stops, and companies pitch their products to treat the symptoms.

Wouldn't you rather treat the problem at its root so you can be freed from its symptoms? After all, no imbalance and no symptoms = happier, clear skin.

Estrogen, progesterone, and testosterone are all naturally occurring hormones in both men and women the same way androgens are. Obviously, men have higher levels of androgens and testosterone and women have higher levels of estrogen and progesterone, but both men and women have all four hormones. When these hormones are knocked out of balance, all sorts of things happen. We get mood swings, we get food cravings, we feel frisky, we feel sad, and we get acne.

As if that's not enough, we are exposed to numerous other external hormones like BPAs in plastic packaging, hormones in the medications we take (birth control, corticosteroids, and lithium to name a few), phytoestrogens in the products we use on our faces and growth hormones in the foods we eat.

Women: It may be the case that you have elevated levels of male hormones, such as androgens and testosterone. Indicators of this may also include hair growth on the face, decreased breast size, increased muscle mass and deepening of the voice. If you think that may be the case, it is best to talk to your doctor and have your blood tested for elevated levels of testosterone. Treating your hormonal problem will help your acne.

Estrogen is one of the most potent anti-acne molecules in the female body. It off-sets too high testosterone levels in the blood and soothes and balances the skin. This is why in the week before your period, when your estrogen levels drop you see acne flare ups.

Progesterone can also play a role in your skin, which I saw first-hand taking progesterone only birth control pills. I had horrendous breakouts and was generally a maniac. In high doses, progesterone acts as in inflammatory agent.

This hormone is at its peak in the days before your period. Aha. That makes sense. This cycle of estrogen dips, progesterone and testosterone surges are normal and healthy, but when taken to the extreme, we see more severe acne, and not just once a month.

Men: You may be over-producing testosterone and androgens. That's why in your teenage years, or even into early adulthood you've seen the most severe acne flare ups. That surge in hormones causes an imbalance which is seen by oily skin and breakouts. Steroid use has also been shown to cause acne along with other really nasty side effects. You don't need me to tell you that steroids are bad news.

Here's what you can do about it:

- Limit stress. Women: whenever your body is under any amount of stress, it decides whether to produce normal sex hormones (estrogen, progesterone) or if it wants to produce stress hormones like DHEA-S, one type of androgen that is responsible for oil production. You see where that leads.

- Evening primrose oil supplements are great for women because they help to regulate hormones. It's been one of the biggest helpers in clearing my skin and calming my serious PMS related mood swings, cravings, and breakouts.

- *Bonus! It's not just for women. Men can also benefit from evening primrose oil's high concentration of gamma linoleic acid, an Omega-7 fatty acid great for reducing inflammation in the body.*

- Avoid High Omega-6 Polyunsaturated Fats. These things are man-made fats found in foods like vegetable oil, canola oil, shortening, fast food, and general junk food. They are highly unstable compounds that oxidize very easily within the body, causing mutation and inflammation of cells.

- Cut back on the caffeine. Hard to do, I know. I love my lattes as much as the next person. Truth is, if you overdo it, it can put undue stress on the endocrine system. Bad news.

- Avoid toxins. They are everywhere, so knowing what you are exposing yourself to on a daily basis can help eliminate a huge chunk of them. Things like plastic packaging, household cleaners, pesticides, non-stick and teflon pans, some lotions and soaps, and even some of those sauces and spices you love contain MSG and toxins that can mimic your body's natural hormones and keep you from producing the ones you need.

- Get your sleep. 'Nuff said. You've heard it before.
- Be picky about your supplements. Not all of those herbs and pills are filling in the gaps, and some of them do more harm than good. You could have a number of deficiencies.
- Do your research, take your vitamins and eat a good diet with lots of variety. Make sure you're getting enough zinc, magnesium, and selenium, as a deficit of those have been linked to acne.
- Get moving. You already know you should. Your body was built to move. Give it what it wants, and it will return the favor.
- **Eat real food.** Your body needs the fuel that keeps it healthy and working in top condition.

Now that you know how to get a handle on your hormones, it's time to evaluate your gut health.

Your gut affects your brain, your mood, your skin, and general health, so it's important to remember this often overlooked area when addressing health concerns.

Make sure you're cultivating healthy gut-flora by consuming enough probiotic cultures like those found in yogurt and fermented foods. They help to kill off the harmful bacteria and replenish the healthy ones that keep your skin clear, your digestion moving, and your brain in top shape.

If you struggle with acne, it's important to see a doctor and run some tests to ensure you have a healthy stomach and digestive system. Issues like candida, leaky gut, and small intestinal bacterial overgrowth can sabotage your overall health.

Please keep in mind that contrary to popular belief, antibiotics are not the answer. They kill the good bacteria that keep the bad ones in check making it easy for bad bacteria to grow out of control.

Also know that infections like candida feed on sugar. Not only is cutting out sugar amazingly good for you, but it also may help clear up candida altogether, when combined with other food medicines like fermented cod liver oil and coconut oil.

Since everyone's body chemistry is different, it's very possible that addressing the health of your gut may be the single key to unlocking your best skin ever. It may be the one thing holding you back.

Clearing our skin is not an exact science, but a process of elimination to figure out what in the body is causing us to breakout.

This guide is intended to be used as a tool to narrow down the potential causes of acne. Because everyone's body is different, what works for one person may not work for the next.

By listening to your body's cues and eliminating

chemical cleansers and toxic products used in your daily life, while adopting healthier eating habits, you should notice improvements in your skin.

While it is my most sincere hope that using this guide has dramatically cleared your skin and helped you feel happier and confident in your skin, please use caution when making dramatic changes, because again, you know your body better than anyone else.

As you commit to making these changes and addressing areas of your life that were not serving you best, you'll notice that not only will your skin change, but your outlook will too.

In this way, I am hoping that you become more happy and see all the beauty and joy life has to offer you. You can be free from acne, you just have to decide it is possible. Make that choice and change your life. You so deserve it.

Best wishes to you on your journey to holistic healing and skin freedom!

Bonus Tips

Maintain Your Clear Skin and Fade Post Acne Marks

Congratulations! You've made it a full thirty days without washing your face! How does it feel? It should be balanced, fresh and healing.

To ensure your skin stays on the path of regeneration, it's important that you continue to avoid conventional commercial cleansers.

It's perfectly fine to rinse your face with water once a day, even twice if your situation calls for it.

When you need something with a little more power, or your skin simply needs a treat, try one of these natural remedies below.

Only choose one treatment a week to reap the benefits of these treatments.

Nutmeg and honey face mask

Mix in a small nonmetal bowl: 1 tbsp raw manuka honey with 1/8th tsp nutmeg. Gently spread this over your face and neck. Leave on for up to 10 minutes and rinse well with lukewarm water. Pat dry. This is an excellent way to fade the post acne marks and kill bad bacteria.

Avocado face mask

Cut up an avocado, mash it and apply it to your face for 15 minutes. Rinse with tepid water and pat dry. Your skin should feel super soft and smooth.

Papaya face mask

Cut a slice of ripe papaya, remove the pulp and rub the peel over your face and neck. Let it dry for 15-20 minutes. Rinse well with lukewarm water and pat dry. The enzymes in the papaya exfoliate, reduce the appearance of spots, help to repair sun damage, and smooth the texture of your skin. Your skin will look brighter with a smoother texture.

Oil cleanser

2 tsp olive or jojoba oil. Rub over your face gently and rinse with a wet washcloth.

Apple cider vinegar & honey face mask

1tbsp acv, 2 tbsp honey: Apply to a clean face and leave on for 20 minutes. Rinse with tepid water. Moisturizes and balances the pH of the skin. Heals post acne marks

Creamy face mask

2 tbsp sour cream (not fat free) 2 tbsp honey and 1 tbsp acv. Leave on for 20 minutes. Heals, exfoliates, brightens, prevents breakouts, moisturizes skin, fades acne marks.

Raw egg yolk or egg white mask

Separate egg yolk and apply either to the face. Leave on for 30 minutes, then rinse well. This treatment tightens and shrinks large pores and really helps to decrease puffiness under the eyes. It's great for excessively oily skin too.

Grape fading treatment

Cut in half green grapes and rub over face. Rinse after 5 minutes. This is great for evening your skin tone and fading acne scars.

Moisturizing banana anti-aging treatment

Mash an overripe banana and spread onto face. Rinse after 15-30 minutes.